The Patient Renfield

by

Mark Madoff

PULP PRESS
VANCOUVER

THIS IS A PULP BOOK

Published by Pulp Press
Box 48806 Stn Bental
Vancouver Canada

ISBN 0-88978-016-1

Frontispiece & Cover illustration by Brian Wert

PRINTED IN CANADA

The Patient Renfield

— Contents —

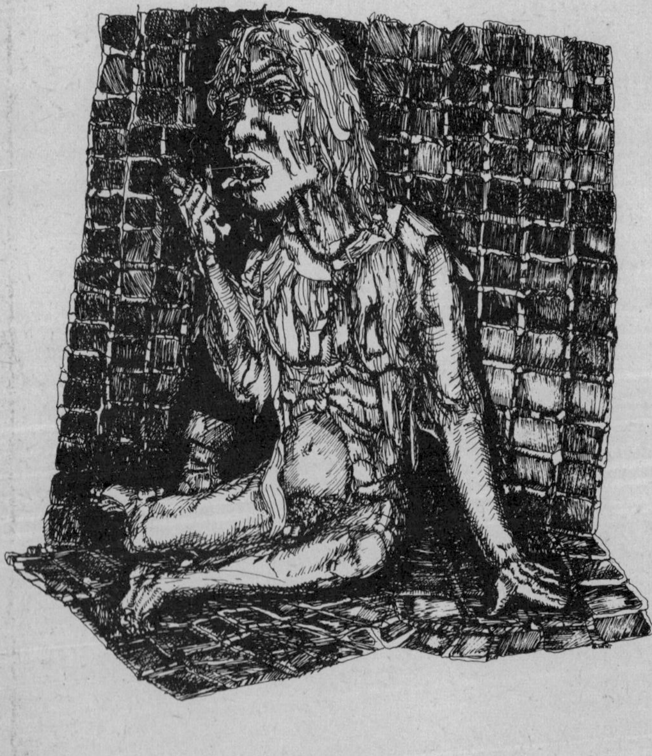

The patient Renfield is crushed to death by his neighbour Count Dracula, who has just entered Dr. John Seward's London Asylum. He arrives through Renfield's cell against which he throws the poor meateater, hard. In his exposition of vampirology, the famous Dr. Van Helsing records that the monster cannot come into an occupied home without invitation.

prayer

O master
send that mist
finer than the nets of reason

o master
come in mist
a drop through the sieve of reasons

o master
drop out your net
sharper than the mist of reason

master of nets
and the mist
of the flow
in the net
in the earth
o master send them

down through proof who stood
me here
like a broom with
my head in the water

clog

The blue fly likes my shits the best
blue fly likes my shit the best
and blue fly likes my shit the best
doctor gives him sugar

and the doctor sends down
rinds from the custardpots
the stiff cud of blancmange
his molasses stillage

i can guess the gall i'd be
if i set on her heels
his goddess of hygiene

if i made him recall what the mutts do
and what the blue flies do
the green and copper too
on his lawn and borders

if i made him recall that even
his own scented stuff
doesn't sift
from his pale closet
to bigger closets

and bigger
if i put it in his mouth

that there is eating somewhere

there is eating in the ground
master of nets

if i carried up to his study
on the dry floor there

my puzzle where they make their puzzles
with the lines drawn all ways
from our lives
jigged
in the cells

my puzzle
why he gives candy to the flies
and the cart comes by

what they do with it
into what hole
in the ground or the river

whose hunger it satisfies

and not my own

experimental entry

I fixed this green fly
on a thorn of paint
the small snot its belly
bibbled the waterwitch
witch in the floor
i was looking for
the lipfeathers sucking all ways
maybe thrown off the joint
and suck a bubble around him

then i laid down the fly on his back
in the brown light by the windowsill

when i pulled off a wing
witching enfolded the whole cell
i was sure it was rich
and i ate that wing

with the next wing
a fizz
tore in the stone edge
he beat over and over
beneath his legs

the eyes the dullest part on the body
and i ate that wing
i was looking for

along the waterline
the light cast down itself
only translucent

the dull body like a blib
of the stone edge

and i ate that thing too

food chains

Keeper can't bring me enough meals in the day
    miss my feed at night
he'll thunk my belly hard at daybreak

keeper can't tell me enough about the feed
    the killers and cutters
the man who does the shopping

those who plow trenches
  to lead the blood from the slaughterhouse
    into the sawdust and ground

those who plant pigshit
  to grow feed to plant
    pigshit

those cats on the yard and behind the greengrocers
  smugly took off the dogs noses
    slapped their eyes white
   their backs after repose
    like the pyramids of feeding beneath them

those who pluck cocks for fishlures
  who hamstring deer for snares
  who wear falcons

those who make soap
pillows candles leather clothing
silk horn handles lacquer
shell kaleidoscopes sera
wigs of real human hair
wigs of real dog hair
artists brushes
classic piano keys
deerhoof bottleopeners
precious objects
subjects for vivisection
many wild railroad victims

trained by the doctor
in recording
the keeper holds these lines for me
like my hat and belt
until sickness passes
thinking now it will pass sooner

turning leaves of the black notebook
he licks his fingers

the language of Daniel

1

In his cell
the patient learns mostly
what the doctor teaches

him and his
mind becomes an ear
a sand castle dug

in the softest
rock the animal ear
at that depth is ready

for a mouth
was coming a dark fist
with no bone shows the

way the head
lies or the hair on the
eye the beard nostril

hole in the
soft sand rock the ear lies
its lips with no

bone in the
hole and his mouth opens agap
when the back turned

sends back
the animal was surring
rock made by it the sand

rock to sand
through the hair is surring
through the doctors face

mouth in the
rock

2

In his cell
the patient learns exactly what
the doctor teaches

so from the start
the doctor told them he wanted
sunday behaviour

with no calendars
with a fleas vista of the brickyard
they didn't have days as such

but they could always have
their sunday behaviour the year
of rice bowls tamping

on the skulls the
shakes drakes gut expurgated
free conversation with the thrill of

listeners on the catwalks
both above and below the wards
sunday behaviour was a whole suit

of shiny clothes
that trust would turn them all
into true sons of their mother

in my reading
i knew exactly what the doctor wanted
for the pious lunatics

were closer
were reweavable they had only one foot
or the other in error

they were also an answer
that the stuffs of science
were not through and through

godless i learned
that with holiness speech could make a year
with the language of Daniel

from the shell
of his castle rock
watched by the lechers of his youth

what i must do to be a better man

1

ABSORB the geometrical
progressions i used
in my work the unconscious copyist
water of this low place
runs in the gravel cone i stood then
fragments unwind like beasts in the coarse paper
each one wrenches in its jaws the tail of one above
now when i learn by grinding what i did then without knowledge
the tide for breeding
for witholding i swallow
i tend
the itching sea
anemone

2

SUCK my own respect
in the body of great enemies
like cannibals i live in a land
without hunger but i believe
in greatness i believe without hunger

and the gorging of livers and lights
takes me over the snow pan to the lee of rocks
cuts the spring river with our own legs
darts the tips fast through great bone

even without hunger in the land
where fruit finds my hand in sleep
and where the reeds rise like breath

only shame lets those lives drop through the net

escaped from shame
i believe in my extension
that i have the care of souls

3

PREY only on predators
the most active and vilest
who choose to gag down
the parts that are undying

the pelts of beasts eaten
spurt in the killers hair
light of the eyes eaten
burns rough stars in their skin

voices plunge through the bitten throat
drift in their shanks like sticky snow
so the killers voice is made
from the clamour in that snow dropping

and they can call anything

like the shrew
like the city of ants
i must feed always

fear of the deaths edge
whacks at my gut like a strop

like a shrew
i must feed always

on nothing less than shrews

visiting day

The doctor comes in with four people
they are wearing street clothes
in a new strange style
the doctor hasn't shown us in the ads

while i watch them fit in the cell
away from the watchholes
where this is spoiling someone's lunch

i think i've been here so long
the streets are named after new dead queens
and my family has forgotten
what it was i should have been doing
and do this here instead

the four look around at me
like angels he just recruited
the grizzly old angel has hips
that could haul a harrow
but he considers my place

unlike the others
he isn't fixed suddenly
by mortar and the brown stones number
or the cleanness of his clothes

he isn't embarassed that he's here
but he seems embarassed that i'm here

that instead of my slavering ink
or rolling my eyes and ears in opposite directions
or counting backward from the year of prophecy

that instead i stand by my cot
with my clean hand out
and say without a quiver
although i rarely get the first word
you are the famous doctor

van helsing and shake his mealy hand
all the time looking as if
i was merely interrupted once
chasing the fixed idea under my tongue

which i'm only waiting here
for my clothes to swallow

the men push ahead their smiles of horror
i name all their aunts and jumping horses

the woman pushes ahead her hand
for me to pluck out the fortune that
makes her eyes so close and wet

the giant check of the old man's suit
hangs in his body a butchers chart
they want me to press against them

my boxes of spiders and flies and sparrows
my little cats and the blue book of notches
they are waiting for me to crack open

this shoestore calm embarassment
to turn around with my seveninch shiv
as the sudden knacker of Smithfield

and they believe this has not happened

already i have jerked each one up
with the nose bursting bloody

already i have guessed right that the texans
thighs are leaner than the english

and the rust is seeping down my hands
from the carrying buckets and spouts and more blades

and the fat old angel has gummed
his beard like dirty mutton

they believe this has not happened

Prey only on predators
the most active and vilest

the keepers joke

But the trees eat rock as well
with their cynics feet
stroking the rock hair

and keeper has the sense
of humour of a vegetarian
that is slow and waterfed

from the smug magic
of percolation hangs down
death in my body

he spread those wide arms
like a poplar wading the flood river

and when he laughs the scales
shake from my back
and turn the laughing stems
screw out my nerve
and screw it in

in this humour
he sent down
butcher blood and blood gravy

but my face in the lid
when they shaved me twice
my thighs in bed and the hair
were like old soap

he also spared whole
loaves of bread and of fat

but my skin still became porous

he also made the cook
set aside his innards
those of the mice once
which he mistook for their potency

but i can only walk the
circuit on his arm
then i forgot how to walk
through walls or how to kill
men without tools

he also loaned me
a bible which he called
the dogs book in honour
of my worship and he wanted
to know for his own sake
which of the prophets was
right about his person and how

their stench was still
buried in this country
and rose like a veil in my gullet

but i told him i heard
nothing by morning or night now
except the tremble of the silver
net of ribbons beneath the cell stones

i don't hear that holy noise from either
face of the cold altar

he also refused me no food
that was my fit he left me
the red bank of the river
which divides the heat in the ground

but my eyes were soon
boils without shadow from it
and the trees there had dried
laughing at the poison of eating

the lion school

When i was a kid
there was no lion school

there was a garden of warriors

even in summer we went to bed early
while they drank gin together

with stones in their mouths

the Royal Menagerie
all the zoos denied
there was a lion school

to start up the lion school
was beneath them

it wasn't what people came to see

in fact the beasts ate only
what could not keep them alive

people came to see the tigers
snatter at nuts but eat them anyway

other times they lay like dry rugs

or lamps if they were owls
hanging in the fatigue of daylight

and the cats licked off their cages

But there has been a lion school
in the great defile
beyond the gasworks

where the trainer roars at their muzzles
until they're greased with spittle

and with his blue arms he pelts them
so they will stop licking smiles and gentleness

he provokes fights among them
by rubbing tiger dung on their arses
but refuses to let them waste their teeth

he has devised the plan for driving
goats against the wire fences
to puzzle the suburbs at the savage hanging meat

his first right at a meal is unchallenged
for he himself has torn throats
and hamstrung

when he is bored with them at last
he leads them down to the common road

there he turns them out
as the different kinds of teeth

as the diseases of joy
and accident and fatality

as the one thin dome of ice
as the unretractable question
whose shadow freezes out the ground

as the allure of pits in the water
and the breaking of children

and the black street with one light
as the dream of losing my eyes

as pillars on the sky
as near animals their fears suddenly exhausted

and the smell of exhaustion
as the minds lice and its picking at them

without this training in blue arms

the world would be infested
with safety

to Count Dracula in the neighbouring ground concerning the dream of appetite

I suffer infinite pity for myself
    beginning as i did here
with my own death in the body
    to relieve my body itself
grown piecemeal on the exhumers
    fork that grubs through luck
through the passes among rock
    finding two bones that talk
when they clack together
    having to try out tongues
like keys in a lock also not finished
    one jaw herbivore
one jaw carnivore
    but the tongue that will eat
everything

    i'm pulling teeth in my hand
i lay out
    shreds the same dream eats
me sleeping stretched
    in a slightly new contortion
maybe my arms are pinned by the belly

    those jaws are still insoluble
this is not like your dream
    of ships timbers and the danger
that is always green

there is a picnic in the valley
    with steep sides
how did any of us get here without falling
    but the grass is so rich and thick
the earth is gone among the blades
    we cut bread there were also meat pies
in the hampers noticing the shape
    of the place we started to eat
above us the day was clear as an eye
    the order of courses was forgotten
it was a picnic the children turned over
    empty baskets and caught dogs behind
the bushes it was so clear
    there were hundreds of us and we kept
on eating some of the people
    were shy and took off their clothes
to chew buttons and hooks and eyes
    later this made it easier to lose
their shyness a man turned a boy
    over an empty hamper
that was added to the big fire
    i saw and ate myself
while the day stood clear over us

    two blue linen napkins
a boys breast and ear
    sardines in hot red sauce
the key
    a squinting mans hair
and my own lips
    that were speechless
from the fervor of grubs
    chattered on a fresh tree
with a whole life like this ahead
    to gag through my mouth and my fat tail
it was hard to walk around with that eating
    among us we noticed the shape
that had come up
    untrue whole bones we walked
hewn without falling like a cursed forest
    transformed in the plague of the ground

the day was clear
    as an eye the wind set over us

one last kiss

Kiss me

no one will hear the truth

count the faces
  lifting my face

count the fingers
  bursting off my nails

count the voices
  barking like vomit in my voice

count the rife blood
  rainbow of the world

you don't kiss me

you kiss the
shit fly
fly spider
spider sparrow
sparrow rat
rat cat
cat rat
rat gull
gull herring
herring hawk
hawk archer
archer bear
bear wolf
wolf gunner
gunner gunner
gunner tree
tree spider
spider fly
fly shit
shit fly
fly spider
spider sparrow
sparrow rat
rat cat
cat rat
rat gull
gull herring
herring hawk
hawk archer
archer bear
bear wolf
wolf gunner
gunner gunner
gunner tree
tree spider

PULP CONTENT

No.1. **The Destruction of Vancouver** by Roy Stone. 75¢

No.2. **The Psychology of the Anarchist** (The Anarchist Peril) by Augustin Hamon. Translated by Jean-Paul Cortane 25¢

No.3. **Lust Lodge** by Rick Torch. 75¢ (bagged)

No.4. **Ubu Rex** by Alfred Jarry. Translated by David Copelin $1.00

No.5. **Duet for a Schizophrenic** by Chris Johnson 75¢

No.6. **Paper Nautilus** by Mark Madoff 75¢

No.7. **Brother Ignatius of Mary** by Mark Young 50¢

No.8. **Crimes, or I'm Sorry, Sir, but We Do Not Sell Handguns to Junkies** by Vicar Vicars $1.00

No.9. **Minimanual of the Urban Guerilla** by Carlos Marighella 75¢

No.10. **The Epic of Gilgamesh as Commissioned by Morgan** by John Kula 75¢

No.11. **Whetstone Almanac** by Charles Tidler 75¢

No.12. **Incest: Breaking the Tabu** by Bill Hall $1.00

No.13. **The Workingman** by Tom Walmsley $1.00

No. 14 **The Patient Renfield** by Mark Madoff $1.00

Mark Madoff was born in Detroit and now lives in Sidney, B.C. His first book of poems appeared in 1973 (*Paper Nautilus*). *Histories of Our Ladies of Burrard* and *Sulphurous Poems* will appear in $3 PULP.